Paleo Down South Cookbook

50 Quick and Easy Comfort Food Recipes

Disclaimer

The author of the book does not contradict any other information found about the game on any other source. This eBook is created for the purpose of helping individuals in learning how to progress in the game. The book is not meant to arouse contradictions. While all the information in the book is authenticated, further information can also be obtained from different sources.

Summary

Comfort foods always bring the image of fat-rich, saucy foods, which needless to say are not considered healthy but what if we told you that we have the perfect cookbook for you that can provide you the recipes of delicious and healthy comfort food. Yes, this cookbook right here is for all those foodies who'd like to take a food trip down south while staying on a strict Paleo diet. Here is your dream cookbook!

We have here 50 Paleo recipes including:

1. Sidelines
2. Lunch
3. Dinner
4. Desserts
5. Cocktails

So, are you ready to go pick out your favorite mouth watering southern food?

Contents

Sidelines

Chicken Salad

Serving Size

Serves 2 people

Cooking Time

Preparation time: 10 minutes

Cooking time: 15 minutes

Ingredients

Raw honey – 3 tbsp

Dijon mustard – 4 tbsp

Red onion (diced) – Half

Celery stalks (diced) – 3

Cayenne pepper – Quarter tsp

Garlic powder – Half tsp

Chicken (cooked and shredded) – Half lb

Salt and pepper – For taste

Yellow plantain (peeled and diced) – 1

Coconut oil – 3 tbsp

Garlic cloves (minced) – 1

Preparation Method

1. Heat some coconut oil in a pan and add minced garlic to it.
2. Toss it around for a while and wait for it to turn to golden-brown color.
3. After that add chicken to the pan too and stir it around for a while. You will observe that after a while it will start changing color too.
4. Add salt, pepper, cayenne pepper and garlic powder in the pan too and let the chicken cook at medium heat until it turns crispy.
5. Combine Dijon mustard, red onion, raw honey and celery in a bowl and add fried chicken in it.

6. Mix it properly and serve!

Nutritional Facts

Calories – 688.6

Carbs – 66.4 g

Fat – 39.2 g

Cholesterol – 85 mg

Vegetable Soup

Serving Size

Serves 4 people

Cooking Time

Preparation time: 20 minutes

Cooking time: 30 minutes

Ingredients

Thyme – Half tbsp

Ground red pepper – A pinch

Oregano – 2 tsp

Chicken broth – 2 cups

Cauliflower (chopped) – Half head

Tomatoes (diced) – 1 can

Onion (chopped) – 1

Zucchini (chopped) – 2

Spinach – 1 bag

Coconut oil – 2 tbsp

Chicken breast – 3

Preparation Method

1. Heat oil in a large pot or sauce and add chicken breasts to it.
2. Keep frying it at medium heat until it turns brown, down increase the heat or it might burn.
3. When it's done, take it out in a bowl and set it aside.
4. Heat some coconut oil once again and add oregano, thyme, tomatoes, spinach and ground red pepper in it.
5. Stir it around until tomatoes start releasing their juice and after that add fried chicken, cauliflower and chicken broth in the pot too.
6. Increase the heat and let it boil.
7. Add salt and pepper according to your taste and after 10 minutes transfer it to a serving bowl.
8. Enjoy while it is warm!

Nutritional Facts

Calories – 350

Carbs – 17.3 g

Fat – 18.7 g

Cholesterol – 69.6 mg

Acorn Squash Stuffed

Serving Size

Serves 2 people

Cooking Time

Preparation time: 10 minutes

Cooking time: 40 minutes

Ingredients

Salt and pepper – According to taste

Garlic cloves – 2

Onion (chopped) – Half cup

Sage (fresh) – 2 tbsp

Coconut oil – 1 tbsp

Turkey (nitrite free) – Half cup

Acorn squash – 1

Preparation Method

1. Heat the oven at 400°F.
2. Slice the acorn squash in half by cutting it length wise and then place it on a greased baking dish face down. Let it stay in the oven for 20 to 25 minutes and after that you will see that it has softened.
3. Take it out and keep is aside so that it would cool off.
4. Heat some oil in a pan and add chopped garlic, onion, sage and turkey in it.
5. Stir it around for 5 to 10 minutes.
6. Spoon the center of the acorn squash to make room for the stuffing and then transfer the pan mixture in the center of both squash pieces.
7. Keep it back in the oven and let it bake for another 10 minutes.
8. After that take it out and serve!

Nutritional Facts

Calories – 163.8

Carbs – 15.2 g

Fat – 6.2 g

Cholesterol – 28.4 mg

Caviar – Texas Style!

Serving Size

Serves 4 people

Cooking Time

Preparation time: 20 minutes

Cooking time: 20 minutes

Ingredients

Red bell pepper (seeded and diced) – 1

Black eyes peas (drained and rinsed) – 1 can

Extra virgin olive oil – 2 tbsp

Salt and pepper – According to taste

Italian flat leaf parsley (chopped) – Half cup

Red onion (chopped) – 1

Jalapeno (seeded and diced) – 1

Yellow bell pepper (seeded and diced) – 1

Lemon juice – Squeezed from one lemon

Preparation Method

1. Mix all the chopped vegetables in a bowl.
2. Include extra virgin olive oil and lemon juice in the bowl too and mix it properly.
3. In the last include salt and pepper in the bowl and taste it to make sure it suits your taste buds.
4. Keep it in the refrigerator for about 30 minutes. After that take it out and serve!

Nutritional Facts

Calories – 470

Carbs – 74 g

Fat – 8 g

Cholesterol – 0 mg

Paleo Coleslaw

Serving Size

Serves 4 people

Cooking Time

Preparation time: 20 minutes

Cooking time: 30 minutes

Ingredients

Cabbage – 1

Honey – 2 drops

Onions (shredded) – 2

Carrots (shredded) – 6

Homemade Paleo mayonnaise – As required

Homemade Paleo Mayonnaise

Eggs – 2

Sea salt – 1 tsp

Yellow mustard – 1 tsp

Cayenne pepper – Quarter tsp

Apple cider vinegar – 2 tbsp

Olive oil – 2 cups

Preparation Method

1. First prepare the mayonnaise. Whisk both eggs in a bowl and then transfer it to the food processor along with rest of the ingredients.
2. Run it until everything is properly mixed and you get a smooth even mixture.
3. Now put all the shredded ingredients of coleslaw in a bowl and add Paleo mayonnaise until you get the desired consistency.
4. You can serve it at room temperature or after refrigerating it when it gets cold.

Nutritional Facts

Calories – 130

Carbs – 27 g

Fat – 1.5 g

Cholesterol – 9.3 mg

Flavored Beets

Serving Size

Serves 4 to 6 people

Cooking Time

Preparation time: 20 minutes

Cooking time: 0 minutes

Ingredients

Beets (canned, make sure they are sugar free) – 16 ounces/1 can

Onion (sliced) – 1

Cider vinegar – 3 tbsp

Honey – Quarter tsp

Preparation Method

1. Transfer the canned juice of beets to a saucepan and keep the vegetable aside in a separate bowl.
2. Include vinegar and honey to the sauce pan and bring it to a boil.
3. After boiling, add beets to the saucepan too and let it stay at medium heat for 5 to 10 minutes. Don't overcook them or else they'll get mushy.
4. Remove the pan from the heat and add sliced onions in it.
5. Let it stand at room temperature for about 2 hours and then refrigerate it.
6. Let it stay in the refrigerator for at least 8 hours and then serve!

Nutritional Facts

Calories – 101.9

Carbs – 9.9 g

Fat – 0.1 g

Cholesterol – 16.1 mg

Green Salad

Serving Size

Serves 5 people

Cooking Time

Preparation time: 30 minutes

Cooking time: 2 hours

Ingredients

Ham (cubed) – 4 ounces

Honey – 3 tbsp

Cayenne pepper – 1 tsp

Onion (diced) – 1

Water – 1 cup

Greens (of collards, beets, turnips, dandelion or mustard) – 2 bunches

Preparation Method

1. Separate green leaves from the stems and put them in a large pot.
2. Add rest of the ingredients in the pot too and keep it at medium heat.
3. Let it cook for about 2 hours and then take it out in a serving bowl and serve warm.

Nutritional Facts

Calories – 68.6

Carbs – 9.9 g

Fat – 1.4 g

Cholesterol – 16.1 mg

Sweet Bacon

Serving Size

Serves 4 people

Cooking Time

Preparation time: 5 minutes

Cooking time: 25 minutes

Ingredients

Bacon (sliced) – Quarter lb

Dijon mustard – 1 tbsp

Brown sugar – Half cup

Preparation Method

1. Heat the oven at 400°F.
2. Mix brown sugar and Dijon mustard in a bowl and transfer it to an airtight plastic bag along with bacon slices.
3. Place that plastic bag on a baking dish and let it bake for 20 minutes.
4. After that arrange bacon slices in a serving dish and enjoy!

Nutritional Facts

Calories – 210

Carbs – 18 g

Fat – 4.5 g

Cholesterol – 20 mg

Southern Style Jezebal Sauce

Serving Size

Serves 4 to 6 people

Cooking Time

Preparation time: 10 minutes

Cooking time: 30 minutes

Ingredients

Honey – Quarter cup

Dijon mustard – Half cup

Pineapple cubes – 1 cup

White wine vinegar – 8 tbsp

Horseradish root (fresh) – 1 lb

Kosher salt – 2 ½ tsp

Preparation Method

1. Finely grate horseradish roots and put them in the blender along with rest of the ingredients.

2. Blend them until you get a smooth paste.
3. Refrigerate it for an hour or two and then serve!

Nutritional Facts

Calories – 713.8

Carbs – 179.2 g

Fat – 1.1 g

Cholesterol – 0 mg

Fried Tomatoes

Serving Size

Serves 2 people

Cooking Time

Preparation time: 15 minutes

Cooking time: 22 minutes

Ingredients

Almond flour – 1 cup

Eggs – 2

Green tomatoes- 4

Olive oil – Quarter cup

Preparation Method

1. Cut tomatoes into thick slices.
2. Whisk the eggs and dip tomato slices in it.
3. Then dip the tomato slices in almond flour.
4. Heat some oil in a pan and then add tomato slices to it.
5. Fry them until they turn golden and then serve!

Nutritional Facts

Calories – 368.7

Carbs – 12.9 g

Fat – 32.4 g

Cholesterol – 211.5 mg

Lunch

Roasted Southern Ham

Serving Size

Serves 15 people

Cooking Time

Preparation time: 10 minutes

Cooking time: 1 hour and 30 minutes

Ingredients

Light brown sugar – 1 ½ cups

Granulated sugar – 1 ½ cups

Honey – Quarter cup

Dijon mustard – 1 ½ cups

Ham (boneless) – 1 lb

Preparation Method

1. Take a bowl and mix honey, sugars and mustard in it.
2. With the help of a cooking brush, coat ham with this mixture.
3. Heat the oven at 400°F and bake ham in it for 20 minutes.
4. After that whether it's tender from the center or not. You will see that the mustard coating is turning into a brown sauce, but don't take it out of the oven until it is properly cooked.
5. Serve while it is still warm!

Nutritional Facts

Calories – 97.4

Carbs – 23.7 g

Fat – 0.5 g

Cholesterol – 0 mg

Gumbo with Sea Food

Serving Size

Serves 12 people

Cooking Time

Preparation time: 25 minutes

Cooking time: 35 minutes

Ingredients

Catfish fillet (cubes) – 1 lb

Okra (sliced) – 1 lb

Shrimp (peeled and deveined) – ¾ lb

Cayenne pepper – Quarter tsp

Tomatoes (diced) – 14

Vegetable juice – 46 ounces

Olive oil – 1 tbsp

Garlic cloves (minced) – 3

Green pepper (chopped) – 1

Celery ribs (chopped) – 2

Onion (chopped) – 1

Preparation Method

1. Heat olive oil in a pan and add onion, green pepper, garlic and onion in it. Toss it around for a while until it starts changing color.
2. After that include cayenne pepper, vegetable juice and tomatoes sin the pan too.
3. Reduce the heat to medium and let it cook for 15 to 20 minutes. You will see that all the vegetables have start to release their juice.
4. Add okra slices, catfish and shrimp in the pan too and let it cook for another 10 minutes.
5. When all the ingredients have properly cooked, transfer it to a serving bowl.
6. Serve while it is warm!

Nutritional Facts

Calories – 187.8

Carbs – 22.1 g

Fat – 4.6 g

Cholesterol – 72.9 mg

Southern Chicken Gravy

Serving Size

Serves 4 people

Cooking Time

Preparation time: 15 minutes

Cooking time: 30 minutes

Ingredients

Chicken – 1 lb

Spices – As desired

Pan dripping (from cooked poultry) – 1 cup

Water – 1 cup

Preparation Method

1. Fill a pot with water and add spice sin it. Bring it to a boil and let it stay on medium heat until the chicken properly boils. Your main ingredient isn't chicken, its spicy chicken water.
2. Transfer the chicken water in a roasted pan along with the pan drippings and keep it at medium heat until the mixture properly mixes.
3. Transfer it to a gravy boat and enjoy it with Paleo bread or bun.

Nutritional Facts

Calories – 27

Carbs – 4.4 g

Fat – 0.6 g

Cholesterol – 1.3 mg

Chicken Pecan

Serving Size

Serves 4 people

Cooking Time

Preparation time: 15 minutes

Cooking time: 30 minutes

Ingredients

Pecans (chopped) – 1 cup

Dijon mustard – Quarter cup

Honey – Quarter cup

Chicken breast halves (boneless) – 4

Preparation Method

1. Slice chicken breast into quarter inch pieces and flatten them using a rolling pin.
2. Mix Dijon mustard and honey in a bowl and coat both sides of chicken with this mixture.
3. Next, immerse the chicken pieces in chopped pecans and arrange them in a baking dish.
4. Heat the oven at 350°F and roast for at least half an hour.
5. When it's done, let it cool for a while after taking out and then serve!

Nutritional Facts

Calories – 397.6

Carbs – 22 g

Fat – 23.2 g

Cholesterol – 75.5 mg

Southern Shredded Chicken

Serving Size

Serves 4 people

Cooking Time

Preparation time: 15 minutes

Cooking time: 30 minutes

Ingredients

Mushrooms (sliced) – 2 cups

Green sweet pepper (diced) – 1

Yellow sweet pepper (diced) – 1

Sweet red pepper (diced) – 1

Onion (diced) – 1

Garlic cloves (minced) – 1

Olive oil – Quarter cup

Chicken breasts (skinless and boneless) – 4

Preparation Method

1. Heat some oil in a pan and add minced garlic in it.
2. When it starts turning golden add chicken breasts in the pan too and cook it at medium heat.
3. Add all the peppers and onion too and cover the pan with a lid.
4. After 10 to 15 minutes include sliced mushrooms in the pan too and reduce the heat to low.
5. Wait for the chicken to cool properly and when it's done, transfer it to a serving bowl.

Nutritional Facts

Calories – 376.4

Carbs – 17.2 g

Fat – 20.3 g

Cholesterol – 68.4 mg

Southern Steaks

Serving Size

Serves 4 people

Cooking Time

Preparation time: 5 minutes

Cooking time: 45 minutes

Ingredients

Red onions (halved) – 2

Eggplant (halved lengthwise) – 1

Yellow squash (halved lengthwise) – 1

Zucchini (halved lengthwise) – 1

Beef top sirloin steaks (boneless) – 1 ¼ lb

Steak marinade – Half cup

Barbecue Sauce/Steak Marinade

Lemon juice (fresh) – 2 tbsp

Lemon peel (grated) – 1 tsp

Ground black pepper – Quarter tsp

Summer savory – Quarter tsp

Tarragon (fresh and chopped) – Quarter tsp

Dill (fresh and crushed) – 1 branch

Extra virgin olive oil – Quarter cup

Preparation Method

1. First prepare the steak marinade sauce. Heat some oil in a pan and add pepper, lemon peel and all the herbs in the pan.

2. Let it stand at low heat for 4 to 5 minutes, you don't need to cook it.
3. After that add lemon juice in the pan, stir well and remove the pan from the heat.
4. Wait for it to cool down and then take quarter cup of the sauce and spread it evenly on the steak.
5. Now place the steak in an airtight plastic bag along with all the vegetables. Pour the remaining sauce on the vegetables and then seal the bag.
6. Keep the bag in the refrigerator for 30 minutes.
7. Heat the grill at medium heat and after refrigerating the steak, remove it from the bag and place in on the grill. Grill it, without covering, for about 20 minutes and then add vegetables to the grill as well.
8. When the vegetables to turn crispy and steak is tender take it out in a serving dish and enjoy!

Nutritional Facts

Calories – 393.4

Carbs – 16.6 g

Fat – 23.4 g

Cholesterol – 94.9 mg

Crockpot Barbecue Chicken

Serving Size

Serves 6 to 8 people

Cooking Time

Preparation time: 5 minutes

Cooking time: 6 hours

Ingredients

Red onion (chopped) – 1

Chicken (bone-in) – 3 to 5 lbs

Homemade barbecue sauce (above mentioned recipe) – 1 cup

Preparation Method

1. One by one put all the ingredients in the Crockpot, cover the lid and keep it at low heat for at least 6 hours. Don't forget to check on it every hour, or it might burn.

2. When the chicken is done, transfer it to a serving bowl and enjoy!

Nutritional Facts

Calories – 369.7

Carbs – 13.1 g

Fat – 22.3 g

Cholesterol – 103.5 mg

Cajun Flavored Salmon

Serving Size

Serves 4 people

Cooking Time

Preparation time: 5 minutes

Cooking time: 10 minutes

Ingredients

Cajun spices – Quarter cup

Lemon juice – Quarter cup

Almond butter (melted) – 1 cup

Salmon fillets – 3

Preparation Method

1. Combine melted butter, spices and lemon juice in a bowl.
2. Coat salmon fillets with the bowl mixture via cooking brush or spoon.
3. Heat the oven at 350°F. Keep the fillets on a baking dish and keep the dish in the oven.
4. After 10 to 15 minutes check if the fillets are done, then take it out and serve!

Nutritional Facts

Calories – 535.3

Carbs – 15 g

Fat – 30.1 g

Cholesterol – 124.9 mg

Dinner

Roasted Ginerg-y Chicken

Serving Size

Serves 6 to 8 people

Cooking Time

Preparation time: 15 minutes

Cooking time: 55 minutes

Ingredients

Garlic powder – 1 tbsp

Pepper – 1 tbsp

Onion powder – 1 tbsp

Cayenne pepper – 1 tbsp

Chicken breasts (skinless) – 6 to 7

Ginger (grated) – 1 cup

Green onion (chopped) – 4

Lemon juice – Squeezed from 2 lemons

Apple juice – Half cup

Orange juice – Half cup

Preparation Method

1. Combine orange juice, apple juice and lemon juice in a bowl.
2. Add grated ginger and chopped green onion in the bowl too and mix it.
3. Now wash your chicken pieces and keep them in a shallow baking pan.
4. Pour the bowl juice on top of the chicken pieces and sprinkle garlic powder, all peppers and onion powder on the top.
5. Keep the baking dish in the oven and set it at 350°F.
6. After 15 minutes take it out and check whether it's properly cooked or not.

7. If it's done, take it out in a plate and serve!

Nutritional Facts

Calories – 218.2

Carbs – 20 g

Fat – 3.5 g

Cholesterol – 75.5 mg

Chicken and Cabbage Stew

Serving Size

Serves 10 to 12 people

Cooking Time

Preparation time: 30 minutes

Cooking time: 2 hours

Ingredients

Water – 8 cups

Chicken bouillon cubes – 8

Chicken broth – 2 cups

Potatoes (cubed) – 8

Chicken breasts – 2 pieces

Bacon – 10 slices

Onions – 2

Cabbage – 2 heads

Olive oil – As required

Salt and pepper – For taste

Preparation Method

1. Separate fat from bacon slices and fry them one by one at medium heat, in a pan. When they have turned brown and soft from all the way to the centre, take them out on paper towels so that they can absorb oil.
2. Chop bacon into small pieces.
3. Next shred cabbage and cut onion into thin slices.
4. Peel potatoes and cut them into small cubes. Fry them in pan along with onion slices and cabbage.
5. After 5 minutes add chicken in the pan too. Make sure that the pan is shallow.
6. Stir it around for a while and add rest of the ingredients too.
7. Bring the mixture to a boil and then reduce the heat.
8. Let the pan stay at medium heat until chicken is properly cooked.
9. When it's done, take it out and shred it into small bites.
10. Add the shredded chicken back to the pan and heat the stew mixture until you get the desired consistency.
11. After that transfer it to a serving bowl and enjoy while it is warm!

Nutritional Facts

Calories – 440.6

Carbs – 57.6 g

Fat – 14.5 g

Cholesterol – 34.3 mg

Shrimp Creole

Serving Size

Serves 4 people

Cooking Time

Preparation time: 10 minutes

Cooking time: 25 minutes

Ingredients

Garlic clove (minced) – 1

Celery (chopped) – 2 Stalks

Shrimp (peeled and deveined) – 1 lb

Pepper sauce – Quarter cup

Stewed tomatoes – 15 ounce

Green bell pepper (chopped) – 1

Onion (chopped) – 1

Olive oil – 2 tbsp

Preparation Method

1. Heat oil in a pan and add all the chopped vegetables in it.
2. Fry them until they are soft and then add tomatoes in the pan.
3. Cook the mixture at medium heat for 5 minutes and then add shrimp in the pan too.
4. Cook for another 7 to 8 minutes and make sure that the shrimp is properly cooked.
5. Garnish with the remaining chopped parsley and then serve!

Nutritional Facts

Calories – 172.3

Carbs – 13.1 g

Fat – 2.3 g

Cholesterol – 172.8 mg

Easy-To-Make Jambalaya

Serving Size

Serves 5 people

Cooking Time

Preparation time: 15 minutes

Cooking time: 35 minutes

Ingredients

Garlic clove (chopped) – 1

Celery stalks (chopped) – 3

Onion (chopped) – 1

Smoked sausage (sliced) – 1 lb

Ground beef – 1lb

Stewed tomatoes – 1 cup

Garlic salt – Half tsp

Water – 14 fluid ounces

Preparation Method

1. Place ground beef, onion, garlic, smoked sausage and celery in a large stock pot and heat it at medium heat until beef turns brown.
2. After 10 to 15 minutes include water, garlic salt, tomatoes, and cabbage in the pot too.
3. Bring it to a boil and then reduce the heat.
4. Let it cook for at least half an hour and then transfer it to a serving bowl.
5. Enjoy!

Nutritional Facts

Calories – 871.0

Carbs – 62.6 g

Fat – 49.9 g

Cholesterol – 146.5 mg

Southern Mustard Chicken

Serving Size

Serves 2 people

Cooking Time

Preparation time: 2 minutes

Cooking time: 15 minutes

Ingredients

Honey – 1 tbsp

Dijon mustard – 1/3 cup

Low sodium chicken broth – ¾ cup

Orange juice (fresh) – ¾ cup

Chicken pieces (skinless) – 4

Green onions (sliced) – 2

Trader Joe's Habanero Hot Sauce – 1 tsp

Sea salt and pepper – 1 tsp each

Preparation Method

1. Coat chicken pieces with pepper and salt.
2. Broil chicken pieces for 5 to 10 minutes and you will see that it has turned brown.
3. Take a sauce pan and add orange juice, chicken broth and green onions in it.
4. Boil it for 4 to 5 minutes then include hot pepper sauce, honey and Dijon mustard in the pan.
5. Reduce the heat and cook the sauce until it gets thick.
6. Take out chicken pieces in a serving dish. Top it with the hot pepper sauce and serve!

Nutritional Facts

Calories – 120.7

Carbs – 23.7 g

Fat – 2 g

Cholesterol – 0 mg

Ham Steak

Serving Size

Serves 4 people

Cooking Time

Preparation time: 3 minutes

Cooking time: 15 minutes

Ingredients

Paleo ham steaks – 1 ¼ lbs

Olive oil – As required

Honey – 1 tbsp

Black pepper – Quarter tsp

Preparation Method

1. Take out paleo ham steaks from the packet and place them in a pan after heating some oil in it.
2. Sprinkle black pepper over your steaks and cook both sides properly until they turn brown and are tender from the center.
3. Top steaks with honey and continue cooking them.
4. Flip after a few minutes.
5. When it's done, take it out in plates and enjoy your ham steaks.

Nutritional Facts

Calories – 185.7

Carbs – 3.2 g

Fat – 6 g

Cholesterol – 63.9 mg

Peach Flavored Chicken

Serving Size

Serves 6 to 8 people

Cooking Time

Preparation time: 6 minutes

Cooking time: 40 minutes

Ingredients

Dijon mustard – 2 tbsp

Honey – 2 tbsp

Peach jam – 1 cup

Chicken – 10 pieces

Peach Jam

Lemon juice – Squeezed from half lemon

Vanilla bean – Half

Honey – Half cup

Peaches – 2 lbs

Preparation Method

1. First prepare peach jam by boiling the peaches and then peeling off their skin.
2. Cut them into small pieces and separate their pit from the center and place them in a sauce pan.
3. Slice the vanilla bean all the way to the center and take out its seed, place them in the pot.
4. Add lemon juice and honey to the pan too.
5. Heat the mixture at high heat and after it boils, reduce the heat to medium and let it cook for 45 minutes.
6. When it turns into a thick gooey mass, remove the pan from the heat and take it out in a jar. Refrigerate the jar and use then required.
7. Coming back to the chicken, heat the oven at 425°F.
8. Mix peach jam, Dijon mustard and honey in a sauce pan and boil it.
9. Arrange chicken pieces in a baking pan and pour the boiled sauce over them.
10. Bake it for 25 to 30 minutes and when it's done, take it out and serve!

Nutritional Facts

Calories – 172.8

Carbs – 42.8 g

Fat – 0.1 g

Cholesterol – 0 mg

Southern Meatballs

Serving Size

Serves 4 people

Cooking Time

Preparation time: 5 minutes

Cooking time: 1 hour

Ingredients

Egg – 1

Ground beef – 1 lb

Spices (of your choice) – 3 tbsp

Olive oil – 3 tbsp

Tomato soup (Prepared) – 2 ½ cups

Preparation Method

1. Whisk the eggs and add minced ground beef in it along with the spices.
2. Mix it properly with your hands and roll it in the palm of your hand to form small meatballs.
3. Heat oil in a pan and fry those meatballs in it.
4. Now take out tomato soup in a sauce pan, heat it until it gets thick and then add meatballs in it.
5. After 5 minutes, turn off the heat and serve your meatballs.

Nutritional Facts

Calories – 262.1

Carbs – 0.1 g

Fat – 18.2 g

Cholesterol – 129.9 mg

Southern Greens

Serving Size

Serves 6 people

Cooking Time

Preparation time: 10 minutes

Cooking time: 1 hour

Ingredients

Onion (diced) – 1 cup

Salt pork (diced) – 1 cup

Olive oil – 1 tbsp

Collard green (rinsed) – 2 lbs

White vinegar – 1/3 cup

Water – Half cup

Low sodium chicken broth – 1 cup

Black pepper (cracked) – Half tsp

Red pepper flakes (crushed) – Quarter tsp

Trader Joe's Habanero Hot Sauce – 1 tsp

Preparation Method

1. Heat oil in a large stock pot and add diced salt pork in it.
2. Fry it at medium heat until all the pieces turn brown and crispy.
3. When they are done, take them out in a plate.
4. Now add sliced onion in the pot and toss it around for a while.
5. Then add red pepper flakes, collard greens and black pepper in the pot and cook them at low heat until collard greens turn soft.
6. After 15 to 20 minutes, add chicken broth to the pot too and cover the pot. Let it cook for at least half an hour.
7. After half hour, add vinegar and hot sauce and when it starts thickening, turn off the heat and serve!

Nutritional Facts

Calories – 50

Carbs – 12 g

Fat – 0 g

Cholesterol – 0 mg

Desserts

Southern Strawberries

Serving Size

Serves 2 to 6 people

Cooking Time

Preparation time: 5 minutes

Cooking time: 0 hour

Ingredients

Strawberries (fresh) – 1 lb

Honey – 3 tbsp

Preparation Method

1. Slice the strawberries and place them in a container.
2. Top them with honey and then place the lid of the container.
3. Now shake the container so that the honey and strawberries mix properly.
4. Refrigerate them for two to three hours before serving.

Nutritional Facts

Calories – 30

Carbs – 8 g

Fat – 0 g

Cholesterol – 0 mg

Simple Southern Ambrosia

Serving Size

Serves 12 people

Cooking Time

Preparation time: 30 minutes

Cooking time: 0 hour

Ingredients

Granulated white sugar – 2 tbsp

Maraschino cherries (drained, rinsed and halved) – 1 ½ cups

Coconut (shredded) – 3 cups

Pineapple (chopped) – 3 cups

Orange (seeds removed) – 6 cups

Preparation Method

1. After chopping and shredding the respective ingredients put all of them in a large bowl.
2. Mix them well and refrigerate for 2 to 3 hours.
3. Serve!

Nutritional Facts

Calories – 131.7

Carbs – 18.5 g

Fat – 6.8 g

Cholesterol – 0 mg

Coconut Sweet

Serving Size

Serves 6 people

Cooking Time

Preparation time: 15 minutes

Cooking time: 25 minutes

Ingredients

Lime juice – Squeezed from half lime

Coconut (grated) – 1 lb

Water – 1 cup

Coconut palm sugar – Half lb

Preparation Method

1. Mix coconut palm sugar and water in a sauce pan and heat it at medium heat until it turns into thick syrup.
2. When the syrup loses its liquid-ness, add lime juice and coconut in the pan and let it stand at medium heat for a little while more.
3. Transfer in to a wide bowl and let it cool before eating.

Nutritional Facts

Calories – 471.2

Carbs – 550.8 g

Fat – 292.9 g

Cholesterol – 0 mg

Cake Filling with Figs

Serving Size

Serves 8 people

Cooking Time

Preparation time: 15 minutes

Cooking time: 45 minutes

Ingredients

Orange rind (grated) – Half

Lemon juice – Squeezed from half lemon

Boiled water – Half cup

Arrowroot powder – 2 tbsp

Honey – Half cup

Figs (chopped) – Quarter lb

Preparation Method

1. First of all cook figs until they turn soft. That will take about half an hour.

2. Take a double broiler and mix honey and arrowroot powder in it.
3. Now start adding boiled water in it slowly while stirring it constantly.
4. Let it cook for 15 minutes.
5. Then include cooked figs, orange rind and lemon juice in the honey mixture.
6. Stir it and take it out in a bowl.
7. Let it cool for 10 to 15 minutes and then serve!

Nutritional Facts

Calories – 67.2

Carbs – 17.2 g

Fat – 0 g

Cholesterol – 0 mg

Glazed Pecans

Serving Size

Serves 4 people

Cooking Time

Preparation time: 10 minutes

Cooking time: 0 hour

Ingredients

Pure maple syrup (avoid processed one) – 1 cup

Pecans (toasted and chopped) – Half cup

Olive oil – 1 tbsp

Pecan jam (recipe mentioned above) – 1 cup

Preparation Method

1. Take a saucepan and mix peach jam and maple syrup in it.
2. Heat the mixture at low heat until it starts boiling.
3. Add olive oil in it and stir.
4. Add pecans in the last and after 5 minutes turn off the heat.
5. Take it out in a bowl and enjoy!

Nutritional Facts

Calories – 864.5

Carbs – 214.1 g

Fat – 6.0 g

Cholesterol – 0 mg

Southern Nut Dessert

Serving Size

Serves 6 to 8 people

Cooking Time

Preparation time: 10 minutes

Cooking time: 0 hour

Ingredients

Honey – 3 tbsp

Brazil nuts (grounded) – 1 ½ cups

Preparation Method

1. Take a baking dish/pie plate and combine grounded nuts and honey in it.
2. Keep it in the oven for 10 minutes at 350°F.
3. After that take it out and serve!

Nutritional Facts

Calories – 253.9

Carbs – 10.9 g

Fat – 23.2 g

Cholesterol – 0 mg

Southern Popsicles

Serving Size

Serves 6 to 8 people

Cooking Time

Preparation time: 15 minutes

Cooking time: 5 minutes

Ingredients

Lemon juice – 2 tbsp

Honey – 2 tbsp

Water – Quarter cup

Peach puree (homemade) – 1 cup

Mango puree (homemade) – 1 cup

Popsicle sticks – 6 to 8

Preparation Method

1. Combine fruit purees in a bowl and then add boiled water and honey in it.
2. Mix it well and the add lemon juice in it too.
3. Fill your Popsicle molds with this mixture and insert the sticks in them through the hole.
4. Freeze the molds for 3 to 4 hours.
5. When the mixture is freezes, take it out of the molds and enjoy before it melts.

Nutritional Facts

Calories – 34.1

Carbs – 8.8 g

Fat – 0 g

Cholesterol – 0 mg

Fruit Frenzy

Serving Size

Serves 4 to 5 people

Cooking Time

Preparation time: 10 minutes

Cooking time: 0 hour

Ingredients

Lime zest – 1 lime

Vanilla – Quarter tsp

Lime juice – 23 tbsp

Orange juice (fresh) – half cup

Lemon juice (fresh) – Half cup

Water – 2/3 cup

Honey – 2/3 cup

Orange zest – Half orange

Preparation Method

1. Combine honey and water in a saucepan and bring it to a boil.
2. Remove it from the heat and let it cool.
3. Include all the fruit zests and juice in the honey mixture.
4. Transfer the mixture to an ice cream maker and freeze it according to the instructions mentioned on the box.
5. When you are done with the ice cream making process, serve your fruity dessert!

Nutritional Facts

Calories – 612.9

Carbs – 158.5 g

Fat – 0.5 g

Cholesterol – 0 mg

Southern Bonbons

Serving Size

Serves 4 to 5 people

Cooking Time

Preparation time: 10 minutes

Cooking time: 0 hour

Ingredients

Cinnamon sugar – 1 tsp

Honey – 2 tbsp

Walnuts – 2 cups

Dates (pitted) – Half cup

Fig – Half cup

Raisins – 1 cup

Preparation Method

1. Place all the fruits and nuts in the food processor and pulse them until you get a powdered mixture.
2. Add honey too and pulse once again.
3. Now take it out in a bowl and roll a small quantity of the mixture on the palm of your hand to form small balls.
4. Roll those balls in cinnamon sugar and serve!

Nutritional Facts

Calories – 22.9

Carbs – 153.5 g

Fat – 0 g

Cholesterol – 236.6 mg

Cocktails

Southern Classic Cocktail

Serving Size

Serves 4 people

Cooking Time

Preparation time: 5 minutes

Cooking time: 0 hour

Ingredients

Orange juice (fresh) – half cup

Apple juice (fresh and chilled) – 1 cup

Vodka (Bazooka, Boyd and Blair, VuQo or any other Paleo brand) – 1 cup

Preparation Method

1. Combine all three ingredients and then pour them over ice in a glass.
2. Your Southern classic cocktail is ready!

Nutritional Facts

Calories – 290

Carbs – 23 g

Fat – 0 g

Cholesterol – 0 mg

Blackberry Lemonade

Serving Size

Serves 2 people

Cooking Time

Preparation time: 15 minutes

Cooking time: 0 hour

Ingredients

Honey – 1 cup

Lemons – 4

Water – 6 cups

Blackberries – 2 cups

Preparation Method

1. Squeeze out the juice of all lemons and transfer it to the blender along with the blackberries.
2. Blend them until the no solid pieces are left behind.
3. Now start adding water in the blender to achieve your desired consistency.
4. When it's done, take it out in 2 different glasses and enjoy!

Nutritional Facts

Calories – 490

Carbs – 138 g

Fat – 0 g

Cholesterol – 0 mg

Southern Toddy

Serving Size

Serves 1 person

Cooking Time

Preparation time: 5 minutes

Cooking time: 0 hour

Ingredients

Honey – 1 tsp

White grapefruit juice – ¾ cup

Champagne – 1 cup

Preparation Method

1. Whisk together all the ingredients then pour them over ice in a glass, your Southern refreshing drink is ready!

Nutritional Facts

Calories – 180

Carbs – 25.9 g

Fat – 0 g

Cholesterol – 0 mg

Red Roaring Cocktail

Serving Size

Serves 2 people

Cooking Time

Preparation time: 5 minutes

Cooking time: 0 hour

Ingredients

Cranberry juice – 1 ½ quarts

Vodka (Bazooka, Boyd and Blair, VuQo or any other Paleo brand) – 1 cup

Orange juice (fresh) – 6 ounces

Preparation Method

1. Take a plastic container and mix all the ingredients in it.
2. Keep it in the freezer and freeze it until you get the slushy-like consistency.
3. After that transfer it into wine glasses and serve!

Nutritional Facts

Calories – 940

Carbs – 100 g

Fat – 0 g

Cholesterol – 0 mg

Southern Classic Cocktail

Serving Size

Serves 2 people

Cooking Time

Preparation time: 15 minutes

Cooking time: 0 hour

Ingredients

Pineapple juice – 3 ounces

Lemon juice – 1 ounce

Orange juice – 2 ounces

10 Cane rum – 4 ounces

Pomegranate juice – 1 ounce

Grapefruit juice – 1 ounce

Tequila – Quarter ounce

Ice – As required

Preparation Method

1. First combine pomegranate juice, grapefruit juice and tequila in the blender and run them for 2 minutes.
2. Then fill 2 glasses with crushed ice.
3. Combine the remaining ingredients in a shaker and then pour them over ice.
4. Top it with the blender mixture and serve!

Nutritional Facts

Calories – 190

Carbs – 14 g

Fat – 0 g

Cholesterol – 0 mg

Instant Southern Coffee Crush

Serving Size

Serves 1 person

Cooking Time

Preparation time: 5 minutes

Cooking time: 0 hour

Ingredients

Vodka (Bazooka, Boyd and Blair, VuQo or any other Paleo brand) – Half cup

Coffee (prepared and cooled) – Half cup

Instant espresso coffee granules – 1 tsp

Coffee liqueur – Quarter cup

Crushed ice

Preparation Method

1. Take a martini shaker and add all the ingredients in it.
2. Shake it well and then pour it over crushed ice in two different martini glasses.
3. Enjoy!

Nutritional Facts

Calories – 900

Carbs – 45 g

Fat – 0 g

Cholesterol – 0 mg

Milky Southern Drink

Serving Size

Serves 1 person

Cooking Time

Preparation time: 5 minutes

Cooking time: 0 hour

Ingredients

Coffee liqueur – Quarter cup

Vodka (Bazooka, Boyd and Blair, VuQo or any other Paleo brand) – Quarter cup

Coconut or almond milk – ¾ cup

Preparation Method

1. Put all the ingredients in the martini shaker and shake them well.
2. Take it out in your glass, add ice if you like and enjoy!

Nutritional Facts

Calories – 190

Carbs – 26 g

Fat – 0 g

Cholesterol – 0 mg

Southern Fruity Slush

Serving Size

Serves 12 to 24 people

Cooking Time

Preparation time: 15 minutes

Freezing time: 6 to 8 hours

Ingredients

Vodka (Bazooka, Boyd and Blair, VuQo or any other Paleo brand) – 3 cups

Tea bags – 4

Water – 5 cups

Lemonade (fresh and frozen) – 1 cup

Orange juice (fresh and frozen) – 1 cup

Boiling water – 2 cups

Lemon or lime juice – 2 tbsp

Preparation Method

1. Put tea bags in boiling water and let them stand for 10 minutes.
2. After the given time remove the tea bags and start adding rest of the ingredients one by one.
3. Stir them well and then transfer it to a plastic container.
4. Freeze the container for at least 6 hours. It will acquire half frozen-half liquid consistency.
5. Take it out in glasses, put a straw in them and enjoy!

Nutritional Facts

Calories – 181.7

Carbs – 13.2 g

Fat – 0.1 g

Cholesterol – 0 mg

Southern Hurricane Punch

Serving Size

Serves 8 people

Cooking Time

Preparation time: 10 minutes

Cooking time: 0 hour

Ingredients

Orange juice – 1 cup

Red fruit punch (homemade) – 3 cups

Limeade – 1 cup

10 cane rum – 1 cup

Crushed ice – As desired

Preparation Method

1. Combine all the ingredients and pour them over crushed ice in glasses.
2. Serve!

Nutritional Facts

Calories – 168.4

Carbs – 24.1 g

Fat – 0 g

Cholesterol – 0 mg

Southern Sangria

Serving Size

Serves 11 people

Cooking Time

Preparation time: 15 minutes

Cooking time: 0 hour

Ingredients

Raspberries – 1 cup

Lemon (sliced) – 1

White wine – 1 cup

Strawberries (sliced) – 1 cup

Coffee liqueur – Half cup

Orange juice – 2 cups

Orange slice – 1

Cachaca – 1 cup

Ice – As required

Preparation Method

1. Mix all the ingredients along with orange and lemon slices in a large pitcher and refrigerate the pitcher for 2 to 3 hours.
2. When it's sufficiently cold, take it out in glasses and serve!

Nutritional Facts

Calories – 230

Carbs – 18 g

Fat – 0 g

Cholesterol – 0 mg

Homemade Paleo Southern Comfort

Serving Size

Serves 1 person

Cooking Time

Preparation time: 5 minutes

Cooking time: 0 hour

Ingredients

Brandy – Quarter cup

Lime juice – Squeezed from half lime

Peach jam – 1 tbsp

Honey – 1 tbsp

Cachaça – 1/8 cup

Preparation Method

1. Blend all the ingredients and transfer them to a glass bottle.
2. Refrigerate it and use whenever required.

Nutritional Facts

Calories – 140.8

Carbs – 16.1 g

Fat – 0 g

Cholesterol – 0 mg

Watermelon Gulp

Serving Size

Makes 1 watermelon

Cooking Time

Preparation time: 5 minutes

Refrigerating time: 24 hours

Ingredients

Vodka (Bazooka, Boyd and Blair, VuQo or any other Paleo brand) – 1 bottle

Watermelon – 1 whole

Preparation Method

1. Wash watermelon from the outside and create a hole at the top.
2. Now pour the entire vodka through the hole into the watermelon and keep it in the refrigerator.
3. Refrigerate in for an entire day before cutting and devouring it.

Nutritional Facts

Calories – 29.9

Carbs – 341.1 g

Fat – 6.7 g

Cholesterol – 0 mg